The Essential ENT Handbook

Simplified Insights into Ear, Nose, and Throat Care

John H. Rios, MD, FACS
Otolaryngologist and Head & Neck Surgeon

Copyright © 2024 by John H. Rios, MD, FACS

All rights reserved. No part of this book may be reproduced, stored in a retrieval system, or transmitted in any form or by any means—electronic, mechanical, photocopying, recording, or otherwise—without prior written permission from the author, except for brief quotations used in reviews or academic purposes.

Disclaimer: This book, The Essential ENT Handbook: Simplified Insights into Ear, Nose, and Throat Care, is designed to serve as an educational resource for healthcare providers. While every effort has been made to ensure the accuracy and timeliness of the information presented, it is not intended to replace clinical judgment or evidence-based practice guidelines.

Readers are encouraged to critically appraise the information and consult additional resources when making diagnostic or treatment decisions. The author, John H. Rios, MD, FACS, and the publisher accept no responsibility for errors, omissions, or outcomes resulting from the application of this material in clinical practice. Always prioritize individualized patient care and stay informed of advancements in the field.

Preface

The field of otolaryngology, encompassing disorders of the ear, nose, throat, head, and neck, is both vast and intricate. Whether managing common conditions such as sinusitis and ear infections or addressing more complex disorders like head and neck cancers, healthcare providers are tasked with integrating diagnostic precision and therapeutic expertise. This responsibility demands accessible and reliable resources tailored to guide clinical decision-making.

The Essential ENT Handbook: Simplified Insights into Ear, Nose, and Throat Care was created to serve as a practical, concise, and authoritative guide for healthcare professionals navigating this dynamic specialty. This book bridges the gap between foundational knowledge and real-world clinical application, offering simplified yet comprehensive insights into key ENT conditions.

Drawing from years of clinical practice, surgical expertise, and teaching experience, I have crafted this resource to prioritize clarity and relevance. Each chapter is structured to provide:

An overview of common and significant ENT disorders.

Practical diagnostic approaches with a focus on efficiency and accuracy.

Evidence-based treatment strategies that align with current standards of care.

Key pearls and pitfalls for managing patients effectively in diverse healthcare settings.

This handbook is not intended to replace detailed textbooks or specialized resources but to complement them by offering distilled, ready-to-use knowledge for busy clinicians, residents, and students. Whether you are in primary care, emergency medicine, or an ENT specialty practice, this book is designed to support you in delivering optimal patient care.

I am deeply grateful to my patients, who continuously remind me of the profound impact of compassionate and informed medical practice. To my colleagues and mentors, your dedication to advancing the field of otolaryngology has been a source of inspiration. Lastly, to my family, your encouragement and patience made this endeavor possible.

I hope this handbook becomes a valuable tool in your clinical practice, helping you navigate the complexities of ENT care with confidence and precision.

John H. Rios, MD, FACS
Otolaryngologist and Head & Neck Surgeon
2024

Preface
Table of contents

Table of Contents

Cranial Nerve Examination

1. Introduction to Cranial Nerve Examination
Importance in ENT and Neurological Assessments
Efficient Organization for Timely CompletionI'm

2. Cranial Nerve I: Olfactory Nerve
Clinical Assessment of Anosmia and Hyposmia
Common Causes: Viral Damage, Trauma, Tumors

3. Cranial Nerve II: Optic Nerve
Visual Field Testing and Fundoscopy
Pupillary Reaction and Visual Acuity Assessment

4. Cranial Nerves III, IV, and VI: Oculomotor, Trochlear, and Abducens Nerves
Eye Movement Evaluations
Identifying Specific Paralyses and Disorders

5. Cranial Nerve V: Trigeminal Nerve
Sensory Testing of Facial Regions
Corneal Reflex Examination

6. Cranial Nerve VII: Facial Nerve
Assessing Facial Symmetry and Bell's Sign
Tests for Lacrimal Gland Function and Taste

7. Cranial Nerve VIII: Vestibulocochlear Nerve
Hearing and Balance Assessments
Tuning Fork and Vestibular Tests

8. Cranial Nerves IX, X, and XI: Glossopharyngeal, Vagus, and Accessory Nerves
Gag Reflex and Vocal Cord Evaluation

Shoulder Shrugging and Head Rotation Tests

9. Cranial Nerve XII: Hypoglossal Nerve
Tongue Movement Observations

10. Emergency Preparedness and Problem Management
Critical Examination Techniques
Immediate Interventions to Prevent Permanent Damage
Proactive Preparation and Resource Management

11. Fine Needle Aspiration Biopsy (FNAB): A Simplified Approach
Importance in Diagnosing Tumors and Nodules
Required Materials
Step-by-Step Procedure
Nodule Identification, Needle Insertion, and Sample Collection
Slide Preparation and Fixation Techniques
Key Considerations and Practical Insights

Ensuring Sample Adequacy
Avoiding Excessive Blood Contamination
Differentiating Benign and Malignant Lesions
Clinical Documentation and Analysis
Importance of Detailed Patient and Lesion Records
Supporting Accurate Cytological Diagnoses

Chapter 1: Acute Upper Airway Obstruction
1.1 Overview of Upper Airway Obstruction
1.2 Locating the Obstruction
Supraglottic
Laryngeal
Tracheal
Bronchial/Lower Lungs
1.3 Approach to Diagnosis and Management
Initial Assessment
Physical Examination
Auscultation and Palpation
Diagnostic Tools

Emergency Preparedness
1.4 Levels of Obstruction and Associated Stridor
Supra-laryngeal
Laryngeal
Tracheal
1.5 Causes of Upper Airway Obstruction
Supralaryngeal
Supraglottic
Glottic
Neurologic Causes
Subglottic and Tracheal Pathologies
1.6 Investigations and Management of Vocal Cord Paralysis
Unilateral Paralysis
Bilateral Paralysis
1.7 Treatment of Upper Respiratory Obstruction
Airway Clearance
Cricothyroid Puncture
Tracheotomy
Emergency Tracheotomy Technique
1.8 Key Principles of Intervention

Airway Clearance and Management Techniques

Chapter 2: Bleeding from the Airways and Digestive Tract: A Clinical Perspective
2.1 Overview of Spontaneous Bleeding
2.2 Identifying the Bleeding Source
Pulmonary Bleeding
Gastrointestinal Bleeding
2.3 Diagnostic Evaluation
Laboratory Analysis
Stool Examination
Imaging and Clinical Examination
2.4 Management
Pulmonary Hemorrhage Management
Gastrointestinal Bleeding Management
Oesophageal Varices
Variceal Ligation and Portal Hypertension
Emergency Interventions
Temporary Control and Long-term Solutions

Chapter 3: Epistaxis: Comprehensive Overview and Management

1. Introduction

2. Etiology and Presentation
Common Sites of Bleeding
Unilateral vs Bilateral Epistaxis
Diagnostic Approach

3. Management Strategies
Cautery: Methods and Indications
Nasal Packing: Techniques and Considerations
Posterior Packing and Balloon Catheters
Vasoconstrictive Injections
Surgical Interventions

4. Conclusion

Chapter 4: Foreign Bodies: A Comprehensive Analysis of Diagnosis and Management

1. Introduction

2. Foreign Bodies in the Ear
Management Principles and Techniques
Avoiding Complications

3. Foreign Bodies in the Nose
Symptoms and Removal Strategy
Instrumental Extraction Methods

4. Foreign Bodies in the Throat
Diagnosis and Management
Advanced Removal Techniques

5. Foreign Bodies in the Larynx
Emergency Management and Techniques

6. Foreign Bodies in the Trachea and Bronchi
Diagnosis and Removal Strategies

7. Foreign Bodies in the Esophagus
Radiographic Evaluation and Endoscopy

8. Conclusion

Chapter 5: Ear Pain (Otalgia)

1. Introduction

2. Key Considerations
Primary Ear Causes
Referred Pain from Nearby Structures

3. Innervation of the Ear
Cranial Nerve Contributions

4. Clinical Approach to Referred Pain

5. Conclusion

Chapter 6: Otitis: Infections and Inflammations of the Ear

1. Introduction

2. Otitis Externa
Pathophysiology and Causes

Symptoms and Diagnosis
Treatment and Prevention

3. Otitis Media
Types and Causes
Symptoms and Treatment Approaches

4. Mastoiditis and Labyrinthitis
Diagnosis and Management

5. Conclusion

Chapter 7: Vertigo and Dizziness: A Comprehensive Analysis

1. Introduction to Vertigo and Dizziness

2. Mechanisms of Balance and Vertigo
Peripheral vs. Central Sources
Brainstem Integration

3. Clinical Features and Diagnosis
Peripheral Vertigo

Central Vertigo

4. Causes of Peripheral Vertigo
Benign Paroxysmal Positional Vertigo (BPPV)
Meniere's Disease
Ototoxicity
Vestibular Neuronitis

5. Treatment and Rehabilitation
Acute Phase Management
Rehabilitation Exercises
Compensation Process

6. Conclusion

Chapter 8: Deafness or Hearing Loss: A Comprehensive Analysis

1. Introduction to Hearing Loss

2. Classification of Hearing Loss
Mild to Moderate Hearing Loss

Severe Hearing Loss

3. Impact of Hearing Loss on Speech Development
Pre-Linguistic Deafness
Post-Linguistic Deafness

4. Causes of Hearing Loss
Conductive Hearing Loss
Sensorineural Hearing Loss

5. Diagnostic Approach
History and Physical Examination
Tuning Fork Tests
Behavioral Tests

6. Management Strategies
Conductive Hearing Loss Treatments
Sensorineural Hearing Loss Treatments

7. Special Considerations
Congenital and Early-Onset Hearing Loss
Tinnitus Management

8. Conclusion

Chapter 9: Facial Paresis and Paralysis: A Detailed Analysis

1. Introduction to Facial Paresis and Paralysis

2. Common Causes of Facial Paralysis
Idiopathic Bell's Palsy
Iatrogenic Injury
Trauma
Infections and Inflammation
Herpes Zoster and Other Viral Infections

3. Prognosis and Treatment Approaches
Bell's Palsy Prognosis
Herpes Zoster-Related Paralysis
Corticosteroid Therapy
Surgical Intervention

4. Challenges in Management

5. Conclusion

Chapter 10: Nasal Obstruction: A Detailed Overview

1. Introduction to Nasal Obstruction

2. Common Causes of Nasal Obstruction
Alternating Obstruction
Persistent Unilateral Obstruction

3. Conditions Leading to Alternating Obstruction
Allergic Rhinitis
Vasomotor Rhinitis
Viral Rhinitis
Sinusitis

4. Conditions Leading to Persistent Unilateral Obstruction
Nasal Septum Deviation
Foreign Body
Nasal Polyps or Tumors

5. Diagnostic Approach

6. Treatment and Management

7. Conclusion

Chapter 11: Sinusitis: A Comprehensive Analysis

1. Introduction

2. Pathophysiology
Initiation
Formation of a Closed Cavity
Fluid Accumulation
Clinical Symptoms
Chronicity

3. Diagnosis
Imaging
Symptoms

4. Management

Medical Treatment
Antibiotics
Nasal Decongestants
Surgical Intervention
Addressing Dental Abscesses

5. Key Considerations

6. Conclusion

Chapter 12: Comprehensive Analysis of Headaches

1. Misconceptions about Headaches

2. Common Types of Headaches
Idiopathic Headaches
Migraine
Cluster Headaches
Sinus Headaches
Sluder Headaches
Cervical and Tension Headaches

3. Less Common Causes

Hypertension
Neurological Conditions
Structural Abnormalities

4. Diagnostic and Management Considerations
Initial Symptomatic Treatment
Psychological Factors
Imaging and Investigations
Parasitic Infections
Referral

5. Conclusion

Chapter 13: Hoarseness or Dysphonia: Comprehensive Analysis and Case-Based Insights

1. Introduction to Dysphonia

2. Extralaryngeal Causes
Psychogenic Factors
Neurological Impairments
Neuromuscular Disorders

Recurrent Laryngeal Nerve Damage

3. Intralaryngeal Causes
Pubertal Voice Changes
Endocrine Disorders
Inflammatory Conditions
Benign Lesions
Malignancies

4. Differential Diagnosis and Considerations

5. Conclusion and Clinical Recommendations

Chapter 14: Tonsillitis and Adenoids: Comprehensive Overview

1. Introduction to Waldeyer's Ring

2. Inflammation and Hypertrophy

3. Treatment Considerations
Initial Phase (First 3 Days)
Secondary Phase (After 3 Days)

4. Clinical Management of Pharyngitis and Laryngitis
 Introduction
Etiology and Classification
Viral Pharyngitis
Bacterial Pharyngitis
Fungal Pharyngitis
Laryngitis
Clinical Presentation
Symptoms and Signs
 Diagnostic Approaches
Management
Pharmacological Treatments
Supportive Care
Complications and Prognosis

5. Conclusion

Chapter 15: Tumors in the Neck and Thyroid Nodules: Clinical Approach and Management

1. Neck Tumors
Persistent Neck Masses: Diagnosis and Initial Management
Fine-Needle Aspiration Biopsy (FNAB): Technique and Benefits
Role of Cytology in Diagnosis

2. Thyroid Nodules
Clinical Features Suggestive of Malignancy
Diagnostic Investigations: Thyroid Function Tests and Scintigraphy
Fine-Needle Aspiration Biopsy (FNAB) in Nodule Assessment

3. Management Strategies
Observation and Medical Management
Surgical Intervention: Indications and Approaches
Post-Operative Considerations: Thyroid Hormone Replacement

Chapter 16: Nasal Fractures: Diagnosis and Management

1. Diagnosis
Clinical Diagnosis and Imaging
Septal Displacement and Trauma

2. Timing of Intervention
Optimal Timing for Reduction
Risks of Delayed Intervention

3. Septal Hematoma and Its Risks
Identification and Complications
Treatment: Aspiration and Nasal Packing

4. Management of Nasal Fractures
Preparation and Anesthesia
Fracture Reduction Techniques
Stabilization and Post-Procedure Care

5. Key Considerations
Handling Septal Hematomas and Early Intervention

Chapter 17: Dysphagia: Assessment and Management

1. Definition and Significance
Overview of Dysphagia
Underlying Causes and Importance of Evaluation

2. Key Diagnostic Considerations
Differentiating Solids vs. Liquids Difficulty
Sensation of a Lump in the Throat
Painful Swallowing (Odynophagia)

3. Diagnostic Approach for Persistent Dysphagia
Barium Swallow and Endoscopy
Advanced Diagnostic Tools and Imaging

4. Summary
Systematic Approach to Dysphagia Diagnosis

Chapter 18: Language and Speech Challenges in Children: A Clinical Overview

1. Significance of Language in Development
Role of Language in Cognitive and Social Function

2. Speech Development in Children
Typical Milestones and Gender Differences
The Impact of Secretory Otitis Media

3. Delayed Language Development
Diagnostic Considerations for Delayed Speech

4. Components of Verbal Communication
Reception, Perception, Integration, Expression, and Voice

5. Diagnostic Approach
Hearing Assessments and Misconceptions about Tongue Tie

6. Conclusion
Early Identification and Intervention for Speech Delays

Cranial Nerve Examination

Cranial nerve evaluation is integral, particularly in patients presenting with vertigo or neurological symptoms. Efficient organization ensures completion within 5–10 minutes.

1. Olfactory Nerve (I):
Assess for anosmia or hyposmia. Anosmia, distinguished by a lack of smell and diminished food taste, can be confirmed with scent identification tests. Common causes include viral damage, trauma, or rarely, tumors. Hyposmia often relates to nasal obstruction or sinusitis.

2. Optic Nerve (II):
Visual fields are assessed by having the patient focus on the examiner's nose while identifying peripheral finger movements. This is followed by fundoscopy, pupillary

reaction tests, and Snellen chart evaluations for visual acuity.

3. Oculomotor (III), Trochlear (IV), and Abducens (VI) Nerves:
These nerves control eye movements. Testing involves following the examiner's finger to identify paralysis or double vision. Specific signs include:

Abducens nerve paralysis prevents lateral eye movement.

Trochlear nerve paralysis causes difficulty looking downward, impairing tasks like descending stairs.

Oculomotor nerve paralysis affects all other eye muscles, easily identifiable.

4. Trigeminal Nerve (V):
Sensory function is tested on facial regions using cotton wool. Corneal reflex evaluation

involves eliciting a blink response with a cotton strand.

5. Facial Nerve (VII):
Facial symmetry is assessed by observing the patient smiling and closing their eyes. Bell's sign, lacrimal gland function (via Schirmer's test), and taste on the anterior two-thirds of the tongue help localize lesions.

6. Vestibulocochlear Nerve (VIII):
Hearing and balance are evaluated using tuning forks and vestibular tests.

7. Glossopharyngeal (IX), Vagus (X), and Accessory (XI) Nerves:
Examination focuses on gag reflex, vocal cord movement, and palatal elevation. Muscle innervation is checked through shoulder shrugging and head rotation.

8. Hypoglossal Nerve (XII):

Tongue movements, asymmetry, or fasciculations are observed during oral examination.

Emergency Preparedness and Problem Management

Proficiency in examination techniques is essential for managing ENT emergencies. Prompt intervention prevents permanent damage, often requiring immediate action without specialist consultation. Familiarity with complications and pre-considered solutions facilitates effective response under stress. While improvisation may be necessary due to limited resources, preparation minimizes risks. Reflecting on Gaspare Tagliacozzi's principle of "Praeceptor Optimum," preparation remains the cornerstone of effective surgical practice.

Fine Needle Aspiration Biopsy (FNAB): Detailed and Simplified Technique with Evidence-Based Considerations

Materials Required:

Syringe: 10 or 20 mL

Needle: 18-gauge (green)

Microscope slides

Fixative: Alcohol jar or clear hair spray

Step-by-Step Procedure:

1. Prepare the Syringe

Fill the syringe halfway with air before starting.

This aids in creating a vacuum with one hand and facilitates the expulsion of aspirated material onto slides.

2. Identify and Stabilize the Nodule

Use the thumb and index finger of your non-dominant hand to locate and immobilize the target nodule or tumor.

3. Insert the Needle

Penetrate the skin and guide the needle into the center of the nodule.

Fully pull the plunger outward to create a vacuum without detaching it from the syringe.

4. Adjust Needle Position

While maintaining the vacuum, withdraw the needle slightly, redirect it at different angles, and repeat the insertion multiple times to ensure adequate sampling.

5. Release the Vacuum

Gradually allow the plunger to return to its original position halfway down the syringe.

6. Remove and Prepare the Sample

Withdraw the syringe and expel the collected material onto a microscope slide.

Cover the material with a second slide, gently pressing them together to create a smear.

Immediately fix the slides by immersing them in alcohol or spraying with clear hair spray.

7. Repeat if Necessary

Create additional slides with any remaining material. Prepare at least three slides to optimize sample adequacy.

8. Send Samples for Analysis

Place alcohol-fixed slides in a secure jar for transport to a pathologist or cytologist.

If using hair spray for fixation, roll the slides in clean paper to prevent sticking and mail them to a reliable laboratory, including detailed clinical information for accurate interpretation.

Key Considerations:

Sample Adequacy:

Visually inspect the sample for sufficient cellular material. Insufficient samples often result in inconclusive cytology reports, necessitating a repeat procedure.

Avoid Excessive Blood:

Excessive blood in the aspirate can compromise sample quality. If noted, repeat the puncture with better control.

Tissue Characteristics:

Malignant tumors with looser stroma are generally easier to aspirate, whereas benign lesions such as lipomas may require additional effort.

Clinical Documentation:

Include comprehensive clinical details about the patient and lesion to support cytological analysis and improve diagnostic accuracy.

Practical Insights:

With consistent practice, operators can assess sample adequacy macroscopically, reducing the likelihood of inadequate results. Proper technique enhances diagnostic yields, particularly in differentiating benign from malignant lesions, and minimizes the need for repeat procedures.

Chapter 1
Acute Upper Airway Obstruction

Upper airway obstruction represents one of the most critical medical emergencies due to its potential to rapidly cause unconsciousness within five minutes and irreversible brain damage in ten minutes if untreated. Prompt and precise intervention is essential, as delays can result in catastrophic outcomes. Physicians must be equipped with the knowledge and skills to diagnose and manage these emergencies effectively.

Locating the Obstruction

The primary challenge in managing airway obstruction is identifying its precise location. The obstruction may occur at various levels, such as:

Supraglottic: Above the vocal cords

Laryngeal: At the level of the vocal cords

Tracheal: In the trachea, either cervical or thoracic

Bronchial or lower lungs: Rarely, issues such as pulmonary edema or pneumothorax can mimic obstruction.

Approach to Diagnosis and Management

Given the life-threatening nature of upper airway obstruction, clinicians must act swiftly with limited diagnostic resources. Key steps include:

Initial Assessment

1. Rapid History Taking: Focus on onset, duration, and progression of symptoms.

Check for prior intubation, foreign body aspiration, or history of allergic reactions.

2. Physical Examination:

Listen to the patient's voice for abnormalities, such as a "hot potato" voice indicative of supraglottic swelling.

Observe for visible signs like nasal flaring, retractions, cyanosis, or tachypnea.

Inspect the oral cavity, mandible, and tongue for trauma or obstruction.

Auscultation and Palpation

Auscultation: Identify stridor (a key symptom), which may be:

Inspiratory: Suggesting supraglottic or supralaryngeal obstruction.

Expiratory: Indicative of intrathoracic tracheal obstruction.

Biphasic: Common in glottic, subglottic, or cervical tracheal obstructions.

Palpation: Examine the floor of the mouth, neck, trachea, and larynx for deviations, crepitations, or masses.

Diagnostic Tools

Imaging: Plain anterior-posterior and lateral neck and chest X-rays are essential. If accessible, fiber-optic endoscopy may be used to evaluate the larynx.

Additional Tests: Blood gases and pulmonary function tests may be performed for further assessment.

Emergency Preparedness

The patient must be continuously monitored until a definitive diagnosis is made. Emergency equipment, including a tracheotomy set, should always be on hand. If airway compromise worsens, endoscopy and potential surgical interventions (intubation or tracheostomy) may be required.

Levels of Obstruction and Associated Stridor

Anatomical Level	Examples of Causes	Strider Type
Supra laryngeal	Nasopharyngeal masses	Inspiratory
Laryngeal	Epiglottitis,	Biphasic

	laryngeal trauma	
Tracheal	Intrathoracic	Expiratory

The upper airway can be divided anatomically for diagnostic purposes:

Causes of Upper Airway Obstruction

Potential causes are classified into congenital, inflammatory, traumatic, immunologic, neoplastic, and miscellaneous categories.

1. Supralaryngeal Obstruction

Congenital: Choanal atresia, Pierre-Robin syndrome

Inflammatory: Ludwig's angina, retropharyngeal abscess

Traumatic: Facial trauma, burns, postoperative swelling

Immunologic: Allergic edema

Neoplastic: Lingual or pharyngeal tumors

Miscellaneous: Obstructive sleep apnea syndrome (OSAS)

Example: In bilateral choanal atresia, neonates struggle to breathe due to an undeveloped mouth-breathing reflex. This condition requires immediate diagnosis and intervention to prevent hypoxia.

2. Supraglottic Obstruction

Congenital: Atresia, laryngomalacia

Inflammatory: Epiglottitis

Traumatic: Surgical edema, burns

Immunologic: Angioneurotic edema, granulomas

Neoplastic: Papillomas, carcinomas

Example: Epiglottitis, often caused by Haemophilus influenzae, presents with a characteristic "hot potato" voice and visible red, swollen epiglottis. Aggressive handling (e.g., using tongue depressors) can precipitate acute obstruction, necessitating careful monitoring and potentially tracheotomy.

3. Glottic Obstruction

Congenital: Webs, atresia

Inflammatory: Croup, laryngitis

Traumatic: Foreign body, laryngeal fracture

Immunologic: Post-intubation granulomas

Neoplastic: Benign or malignant tumors

Example: Viral croup often manifests with a characteristic "barking" cough and biphasic stridor. Treatment includes corticosteroids and nebulized epinephrine.

Neurologic: Vocal Cord Paralysis (Unilateral and Bilateral)

The glottis, a highly mobile structure within the rigid upper airway, serves a critical function primarily for protecting the lungs, with voice production being a secondary, incidental role. Pathologies affecting this region typically manifest as hoarseness, particularly in unilateral vocal cord paralysis, long before stridor develops. Exceptions exist, such as bilateral vocal cord paralysis in adduction, which leads to severe stridor with minimal vocal changes.

Clinical Manifestations and Challenges:

Severe Cases and Atresia:
Complete glottic webs or atresia are life-threatening unless identified and treated immediately after birth. Partial atresia may present as feeding difficulties or aspiration during the neonatal period.

Inflammatory Conditions:
Upper respiratory infections often result in earlier stridor in infants due to their narrower airways. Close monitoring of patients with laryngeal trauma—common in sports or vehicular accidents—is essential, as associated edema can rapidly lead to respiratory insufficiency.

Foreign Body Obstruction:
The glottic level often traps foreign bodies due to its narrow structure and the

protective laryngeal spasm. While the cough reflex generally expels the object, in rare cases, hypoxia can cause the object to move deeper into the airway, necessitating immediate intervention.

Chronic Conditions:
Tuberculosis or prolonged intubation may lead to granulomatous inflammation and subsequent fibrosis. Early medical intervention, including corticosteroids in specific cases such as laryngeal tuberculosis, is crucial to prevent stenosis.

Neoplastic Processes:
Neoplasms at the vocal cord level often present early with hoarseness. Smokers with persistent hoarseness (lasting over six weeks) should undergo prompt evaluation and biopsy to exclude malignancy. In children, laryngeal papilloma, frequently linked to maternal condyloma, poses significant therapeutic challenges, requiring

timely surgical management to minimize complications.

Investigations and Management of Vocal Cord Paralysis:

Unilateral Paralysis:
Typically causes hoarseness without significant respiratory distress except during exertion.

Bilateral Paralysis:
Presents as severe stridor with the vocal cords adducted at the midline, often necessitating an emergency tracheotomy.

In all cases of vocal cord paralysis, thorough evaluation of the recurrent and vagus nerves is imperative to identify the underlying etiology, which may include thyroid surgery complications, cardiac or pulmonary pathologies, or neoplasms.

Subglottic and Tracheal Pathologies

Congenital Disorders:

Stenosis: Narrowing of the tracheal lumen requiring early intervention.

Tracheomalacia: Structural weakness of the tracheal walls.

Inflammatory Conditions:

Laryngo-tracheo-bronchitis (Croup):
A viral inflammation that may involve bacterial superinfection (10-15% of cases), often requiring antibiotics despite diagnostic challenges.

Traumatic and Post-Intubation Complications:

Foreign Bodies:
Usually pass through the glottis to lodge in the main bronchi. Rapid identification and removal are critical.

Post-Intubation Stenosis:
Caused by excessive cuff pressure, resulting in mucosal necrosis and subsequent fibrosis. Progressive stridor is a common presentation.

Neoplastic and Immunological Causes:

Granulomatous Conditions:
Tuberculosis and prolonged intubation may lead to chronic inflammation and fibrosis, necessitating early therapeutic measures.

Tumors:
Laryngeal neoplasms, such as medullary carcinoma, can compress or invade the trachea, causing obstruction.

Treatment of Upper Respiratory Obstruction

Key Principles:

Establishing an airway is paramount, with progression from the least invasive to the most invasive procedures as required:

1. Airway Clearance:
Remove secretions and attempt intubation where feasible.

2. Cricothyroid Puncture:
A temporary emergency measure providing immediate oxygenation.

3. Tracheotomy:
Reserved for critical cases; requires surgical expertise, adequate lighting, and instruments to avoid complications.

Emergency Tracheostomy Technique:

Performed under local anesthesia, the procedure involves:

Extending the patient's neck for optimal exposure.

Palpating the thyroid and cricoid cartilages to guide a horizontal skin incision at the cricoid level.

Dissecting the strap muscles vertically to expose the trachea.

Handling the thyroid isthmus carefully to minimize bleeding.

Creating a controlled entry into the trachea for airway access.

Proper training and anatomical knowledge are essential to minimize risks and ensure successful outcomes.

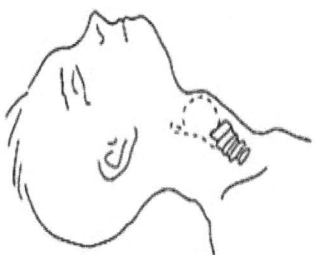

Figure 1

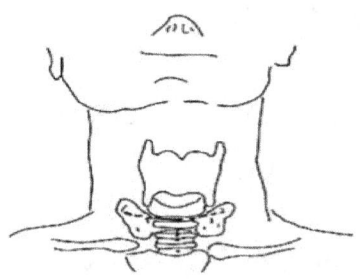

Figure 2

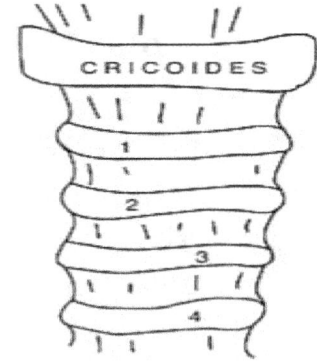

Figure 3

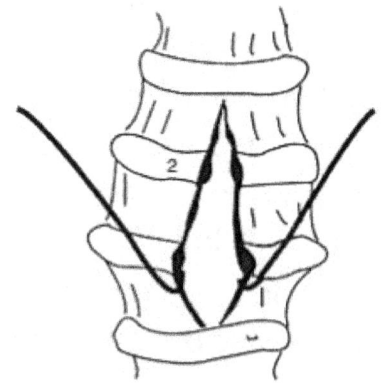

Figure 4

Chapter 2
Bleeding from the Airways and Digestive Tract: A Clinical Perspective

Minor bleeding, such as from the nose or gums, is typically a benign and commonplace occurrence, often not warranting significant concern. Similarly, tuberculosis patients may exhibit minor blood streaks in their sputum without alarm. However, substantial bleeding, such as massive epistaxis, haematemesis (vomiting of blood), or haemoptysis (coughing up blood), constitutes a medical emergency, second only to ensuring a patent airway. This discussion excludes traumatic causes like injuries from knives, gunshots, or accidents, which require distinct interventions. Instead, it focuses on spontaneous bleeding, which can arise from conditions like esophageal varices, gastric ulcers, or erosion of the pulmonary artery due to carcinoma or tuberculosis.

Identifying the Bleeding Source

1. Pulmonary Bleeding

Characterized by bright red, frothy blood and typically linked to severe coughing episodes.

Common causes include tuberculosis or bronchial carcinoma, with tuberculosis patients often having a history of chronic cough or a prior diagnosis.

In bronchial carcinoma, bleeding may be the initial symptom, particularly in older patients with a history of heavy smoking.

2. Gastrointestinal Bleeding

Manifests as haematemesis with dark or fresh blood and "coffee ground" vomitus, indicating bleeding from the oesophagus, stomach, or duodenum.

Some patients may mistake blood exiting through the nasopharynx for epistaxis.

Diagnostic Evaluation

1. Laboratory Analysis

A full blood count (FBC) provides an approximate measure of blood loss. For instance, a drop in haemoglobin by 1g/dL suggests a loss of approximately 500 mL of blood. Significant drops (e.g., from 14 to 10 g/dL) indicate major blood loss (1.5 to 2 liters).

Haemodilution can delay detection of haemoglobin and haematocrit changes for 12–24 hours after acute bleeding.

Immature erythrocytes in peripheral blood may suggest chronic bleeding lasting at least a week.

2. Stool Examination

The presence of melaena (black, tarry stools) is indicative of upper gastrointestinal bleeding and usually develops days after the initial hemorrhage.

3. Imaging and Clinical Examination

Chest auscultation and X-rays are critical for haemoptysis. Persistent bleeding may necessitate emergency thoracotomy and potentially resection of the affected lung segment, especially in curable conditions like tuberculosis.

Endoscopy (bronchoscopy or gastroscopy) can be invaluable for pinpointing bleeding sites, though active hemorrhage may obscure visibility, necessitating reliance on clinical evaluation.

Management

1. Pulmonary Hemorrhage

Pulmonary bleeding caused by advanced bronchial carcinoma may offer limited treatment options, but tuberculosis-related bleeding is curable with appropriate pharmacotherapy.

2. Gastrointestinal Bleeding

Esophageal varices are often associated with portal hypertension and liver dysfunction. Signs include icteric sclerae and a history of hepatitis or alcoholism.

Temporary control of variceal bleeding can be achieved using a balloon catheter, but definitive management involves variceal ligation or reducing portal hypertension via shunt procedures. These interventions carry risks, including exacerbation of hepatic encephalopathy. Liver transplantation remains the ultimate solution for irreversible liver failure.

In life-threatening bleeding, emergency interventions take precedence over diagnostic procedures. Prompt stabilization, identification of the bleeding source, and targeted treatment are essential to improving patient outcomes.

Chapter 3
EPISTAXIS: Comprehensive Overview and Management

Epistaxis, or nosebleed, is a frequent clinical condition, often resolving spontaneously within minutes. However, in certain cases, it can escalate to a critical medical emergency requiring prompt intervention.

Etiology and Presentation

The bleeding can originate from any location within the nasal cavity, most commonly from the nasal septum rather than the lateral wall. It involves either venous or arterial vessels. In younger individuals, the veins in Little's area are typically implicated.

Epistaxis is usually unilateral, stemming from a single vessel, although repeated trauma from nasal packing can create an impression of multiple bleeding points. It is essential to determine the primary site of bleeding, as severe cases may cause blood to flow around the nasal septum through the nasopharynx and exit from the contralateral nostril. This can mislead practitioners into suspecting bilateral bleeding.

A key diagnostic step is asking the patient which side initiated the bleed to guide focused treatment. Initial management involves clearing clotted blood from the nasal cavity, either by aspiration or gentle nasal blowing. A 5 cm cotton pledget soaked in a combination of lidocaine (10%) and a vasoconstrictor (e.g., adrenaline, oxymetazoline) is inserted parallel to the palate. After five minutes, the pledget is removed, and the nasal cavity is examined under adequate lighting. If the bleeding source is visible, it indicates an anterior epistaxis, which is relatively easier to treat. Conversely, an obscured bleeding point may suggest posterior epistaxis, presenting greater challenges.

Management Strategies for Epistaxis

1. Cautery

When the bleeding vessel is identifiable (often as a red, elevated point or a vessel with a visible red ribbon), it can be cauterized using:

Silver nitrate

Trichloroacetic acid

Electrocautery (ensuring nostril protection using IV tubing to shield surrounding tissues).

For cases where these options are unavailable, ribbon gauze packing may be employed.

2. Nasal Packing

Packing is often necessary for uncontrolled bleeding. The procedure involves:

Administering adequate anesthesia to minimize discomfort.

Using a 1-inch ribbon gauze, inserted systematically along the nasal floor (parallel to the palate) to fill the nasal cavity from the bottom upwards. Proper technique avoids loosening of the pack, which may occur if the roof is mistakenly targeted.

Key considerations include:

Monitoring for residual bleeding, as clot contraction within the pack may mimic recurrent hemorrhage. Avoid removing the pack unless active bleeding with clots is observed.

Reviewing the posterior pharyngeal wall to ensure no blood tracking downward.

Advising patients to avoid bending, heavy lifting, and nasal blowing. Sneezing with the mouth open reduces intranasal venous pressure. The pack can generally be removed after 3–4 days.

3. Posterior Packing and Balloon Catheters

For posterior epistaxis, methods include:

Posterior Packing: A gauze roll tied with silk sutures is positioned in the nasopharynx using nasal cannulas passed through the nostrils and pulled out via the mouth. This technique, though effective, is cumbersome and distressing for patients.

Balloon Catheters: A more efficient approach involves using a Foley catheter (#14 or #16). The catheter is inserted into the nose until the tip is visible in the oropharynx. The balloon is inflated with 5–7 mL of air and pulled back to anchor it in the posterior choana. The anterior nose is then tightly packed around the catheter, with tension maintained using a clip to prevent displacement. Antibiotics are prescribed to prevent sinusitis or infections from nasal flora. The balloon and pack are removed after 5 days if no bleeding recurs.

4. Vasoconstrictive Injections

For severe bleeding, injecting 3–5 mL of lignocaine with adrenaline into the pterygopalatine fossa via the greater palatine canal can induce vasoconstriction of the internal maxillary artery, providing up to 30 minutes of hemostasis. This window allows for careful exploration, cauterization, or packing.

5. Surgical Intervention

In refractory cases, surgical ligation of key arteries may be required, particularly in patients with hypertension, cardiovascular disease, or anticoagulant therapy. Techniques include:

Ethmoidal Artery Ligation: Accessed through an orbital incision, the anterior and posterior ethmoidal arteries are identified and ligated or cauterized.

Internal Maxillary Artery Ligation: Performed through a maxillary sinus window, this approach necessitates precise anatomical dissection to clip the vessel.

External Carotid Artery Ligation: Involves a neck incision to isolate and ligate the artery. Familiarity with neck anatomy is critical to avoid complications such as hemiplegia from inadvertent ligation of the internal or common carotid artery.

Conclusion

Effective management of epistaxis relies on accurate diagnosis, appropriate use of packing or cautery, and the judicious application of advanced techniques such as posterior packing, catheter insertion, or surgical ligation. Tailored interventions, guided by the severity and location of bleeding, ensure optimal outcomes and patient safety.

Chapter 4
Foreign Bodies: A Comprehensive Analysis of Diagnosis and Management

Foreign Bodies in the Ear

Foreign bodies lodged in the external auditory canal, particularly in children, are a frequent occurrence. These are often mishandled, causing more harm during removal than the object itself. While their removal is important, it is generally not an emergency unless it causes severe discomfort or external otitis.

Management Principles:

1. Avoid Using Forceps: Using forceps can inadvertently push the object deeper, risking damage to the eardrum or middle ear.

2. Use of Hooks: Small hooks are preferred for extraction. If unavailable, improvised

tools such as bent hairpins or modified needles can be utilized. These should be carefully guided past the foreign body, ensuring the hook catches the object before being gently withdrawn.

3. Irrigation: If space permits, ear syringing with warm, clean water (to prevent vestibular disturbances) can effectively dislodge objects. The syringe stream should be directed towards the ear canal's roof and not directly at the eardrum to avoid perforation.

Foreign Bodies in the Nose

Unilateral nasal discharge in children is highly suggestive of a foreign body. Prompt removal is crucial to prevent aspiration or secondary complications.

Removal Strategy:

Preparation: Clean nasal secretions and apply a topical anesthetic like 10% Lidocaine for pain-free removal.

Immobilization: Children should be held securely, often with the assistance of a caregiver, to prevent sudden movements.

Instrumental Extraction: A small hook or probe should be maneuvered below the foreign body to lift it out of the nostril. Care must be taken to avoid pushing the object deeper into the nasal cavity.

Foreign Bodies in the Throat

Commonly encountered foreign bodies in the throat include fish or chicken bones, which typically lodge between the tonsils and pyriform fossa. These cause pain on swallowing, often persisting since the last meal.

Approach to Removal:

Visual Inspection: Use a laryngeal mirror under adequate lighting to locate the foreign object.

Topical Anesthetic: Spray the throat with 10% Xylocaine to ensure patient cooperation.

Instrumental Removal: Employ forceps (e.g., Tilley's or McGill's) for extraction. Proper orientation using the mirror image requires practice.

Advanced Cases: If removal fails due to patient non-cooperation, a short general anesthetic may be required. Skilled professionals should handle such cases to avoid complications.

Foreign Bodies in the Larynx

Laryngeal foreign bodies often present with stridor and respiratory distress, constituting a medical emergency.

Emergency Management:

Initial Maneuvers: Attempt the Heimlich maneuver to expel the object.

Advanced Techniques: If unsuccessful, direct laryngoscopy under anesthesia is necessary. The object should be carefully retrieved without pushing it further into the airway.

Foreign Bodies in the Trachea and Bronchi

Foreign objects in the trachea or bronchi pose life-threatening risks due to potential airway obstruction. The right bronchus is more commonly affected due to its straighter anatomy.

Diagnosis and Removal:

Initial Symptoms: Violent coughing is followed by an asymptomatic phase until infection or atelectasis develops.

Diagnostic Tools: Flexible bronchoscopy aids in visualization, but rigid bronchoscopy is preferred for large objects. Urological basket catheters may assist in retrieving round or slippery items.

Foreign Bodies in the Esophagus

These objects, often fish bones or meat, cause swallowing difficulties and localized pain. Patients may report attempts to dislodge the object with food, such as bread, with variable success.

Management and Complications:

Radiographic Evaluation: Radiopaque objects are easily identified on X-rays, whereas non-opaque objects may cause air trapping visible on lateral neck or chest X-rays.

Endoscopy: Endoscopy remains the definitive diagnostic and therapeutic tool. However, rigid esophagoscopy, although effective, carries significant risks, including esophageal perforation and subsequent mediastinitis, necessitating expert supervision.

Conclusion

The management of foreign bodies varies depending on the location and associated risks. Proper tools, meticulous techniques, and careful planning are essential to ensure successful removal and minimize complications. Prompt intervention is crucial in emergencies, such as foreign bodies in the airway, while others, like objects in the ear, allow for a more measured approach. Advanced cases should always involve specialists to ensure patient safety and optimal outcomes.

Chapter 5
Ear Pain (Otalgia)

Ear pain, also known as otalgia, warrants a thorough evaluation due to its diverse range of potential causes. Identifying the underlying source requires careful examination, particularly if symptoms such as hearing loss or dizziness accompany the pain, as this often indicates a primary ear condition. If the ear appears normal, attention should shift to surrounding structures, as referred pain is common in otalgia.

Key Considerations

1. Primary Ear Causes

Conduct a meticulous inspection of the ear, from the pinna to the eardrum, using direct visualization and appropriate diagnostic tools.

Functional tests, especially for labyrinthine issues, should assess dizziness or balance disturbances.

2. Referred Pain

Otalgia may result from conditions affecting nearby anatomical structures. For instance:

Tonsillitis frequently refers to pain in the ear.

Temporomandibular joint (TMJ) dysfunction and dental issues may manifest as deep ear pain.

Innervation of the Ear

The ear's complex and overlapping nerve supply necessitates examining various potential pain pathways:

Trigeminal Nerve (Cranial Nerve V): Primarily supplies the external ear canal.

Facial Nerve (Cranial Nerve VII): Although primarily motor, it carries sensory fibers from the tympanic plexus.

Glossopharyngeal Nerve (Cranial Nerve IX): Supplies the middle ear and tympanic plexus via Jacobson's nerve.

Vagus Nerve (Cranial Nerve X): Contributes Arnold's nerve, innervating the posterior external canal, often eliciting a cough reflex when stimulated.

Accessory Nerve (Cranial Nerve XI): Provides fibers to Arnold's nerve.

Cervical Nerves (C2 & C3): Through the greater auricular and lesser occipital nerves, these supply the pinna.

Clinical Approach to Referred Pain

Explore potential sources of referred pain along the nerve pathways mentioned.

Assess for conditions ranging from the skull base to the cervical spine and as far forward as the maxillary sinuses and nasal cavity.

Referred otalgia may arise from pathology anywhere along these nerves, much like how trauma to the elbow can cause tingling in the fingers.

Conclusion

Addressing ear pain involves a dual focus: ruling out primary ear issues and systematically evaluating referred pain sources. By understanding the ear's intricate innervation, clinicians can identify and manage conditions contributing to otalgia effectively.

Chapter 6
Otitis: Infections and Inflammations of the Ear

Ear infections and inflammations are classified into several categories for clarity: otitis , myringitis, otitis media, mastoiditis, and labyrinthitis. These conditions vary in their origin, pathophysiology, and clinical presentation.

Otitis Externa

Otitis affects the outer ear, extending to the eardrum. It is primarily a dermatological issue caused by bacterial invasion of the skin flora. This condition is separate from infections of the middle ear and mastoid, which are typically caused by respiratory tract bacteria. An intact eardrum provides a barrier between these areas, but a perforation can enable resistant skin bacteria to invade the middle ear.

The outer ear canal, being confined by bone and cartilage, allows limited space for inflammation. This restriction often leads to intense pain, especially when the canal swells shut, resulting in a blocked sensation. Symptoms may include pain during movement of the pinna or while chewing, accompanied by a slight, watery discharge mixed with squamous debris.

Factors such as prolonged water exposure during swimming can predispose individuals to otitis by softening and damaging the meatal skin, enabling bacteria to penetrate. Treatment involves cleaning the ear gently with a cotton-tipped probe and administering topical antibiotics, such as ear drops, powders, or antibiotic creams. Acid ear drops (a 50:50 mixture of vinegar and boiled water) may also be effective. In severe cases, filling the ear with broad-spectrum antibiotic ointment using a syringe can provide relief and cure the infection within days.

Necrotizing Otitis Externa

A severe form, necrotizing otitis , primarily affects immunocompromised, diabetic, or elderly patients. Caused by Pseudomonas bacteria, it can rapidly progress to the skull base, leading to severe pain, discharge, and cranial nerve involvement, often starting with facial palsy. Early recognition and aggressive treatment with antibiotics and diabetes management are critical. In advanced cases, surgical debridement may be necessary. Prognosis is poor if the infection spreads to the skull base.

Myringitis

Myringitis, which affects the eardrum, sits at the interface of external and middle ear infections. A specific type, bullous myringitis, involves hemorrhagic bullae on the eardrum, often extending to the external canal. Typically viral, this condition is associated with upper respiratory infections and is characterized by excruciating pain. If the bullae bursts, blood-stained discharge may occur. Treatment is supportive, focusing on pain relief. In rare cases, extensive damage may result in large, non-healing perforations.

Otitis Media

Otitis media is further categorized into acute, secretory, and chronic suppurative types, each with distinct pathophysiology and clinical features:

1. Acute Otitis Media (AOM)
AOM often begins with a viral upper respiratory infection that causes Eustachian tube dysfunction, leading to negative

pressure in the middle ear and subsequent fluid accumulation. This condition can escalate into suppurative otitis media if bacterial infection occurs, resulting in pus formation, drum bulging, and severe pain. Untreated, the drum may perforate, releasing pus and relieving pain. Treatment includes nasal decongestants, antibiotics, and, in severe cases, myringotomy (a controlled incision in the drum to drain pus).

2. Secretory Otitis Media (SOM)
SOM, or "glue ear," involves persistent fluid in the middle ear following an infection, often due to impaired Eustachian tube function. In children, anatomical and immunological factors increase susceptibility. If untreated, the fluid may become thickened and persist for months, causing hearing loss. Management includes monitoring, nasal decongestants, and addressing contributing factors.

3. Chronic Suppurative Otitis Media (CSOM)
CSOM results from recurrent infections through a perforated eardrum. Chronic discharge, often worsened by poor hygiene or water exposure, damages the middle ear mucosa and ossicles. Treatment involves meticulous cleaning, liberal application of antibiotic drops, and maintaining a dry ear. In some cases, surgical intervention may be necessary.

Cholesteatoma

A cholesteatoma is a benign yet destructive epithelial retraction cyst in the middle ear, characterized by progressive damage to ossicles, the mastoid, and potentially the inner ear. Symptoms include conductive hearing loss, vertigo, and foul-smelling discharge due to trapped debris. Untreated, complications such as meningitis may occur. Diagnosis often relies on clinical signs and imaging. Treatment involves surgical removal of the cyst to prevent further complications.

Summary

Ear infections encompass a spectrum of conditions with varying etiologies and severities. Timely and appropriate management, from topical therapies for otitis to surgical intervention for cholesteatoma, is essential to prevent complications and preserve hearing.

Chapter 7
Vertigo and Dizziness: A Comprehensive Analysis

Vertigo and dizziness, while frequently used interchangeably, represent distinct clinical phenomena. Vertigo refers to a sensation of spinning or movement, either of the patient or their surroundings. In contrast, dizziness is a more general term indicating unsteadiness without a clear sense of rotation. While dizziness can result from numerous conditions, true vertigo typically stems from dysfunction in the vestibular pathways or the brainstem. Vertigo can be classified as central (originating in the brainstem or cerebellum) or peripheral (involving the inner ear or vestibular nerve).

Mechanisms of Balance and Vertigo

The brainstem serves as the integration center for signals from the inner ear, visual system, and proprioceptive receptors in the muscles and joints, particularly those in the neck. These inputs collectively enable spatial orientation and postural balance. Understanding whether vertigo arises from a peripheral or central source is critical, as central vertigo generally has a more severe prognosis.

Clinical Features and Diagnosis

The distinction between peripheral and central vertigo can often be made through history-taking and clinical examination:

1. Peripheral Vertigo

Onset: Sudden, episodic, or variable in duration.

Symptoms: May include hearing loss, tinnitus, nausea, vomiting, and marked nystagmus (involuntary eye movements).

Absence of CNS Symptoms: No cranial nerve palsies or other neurological deficits.

Caloric Test: Reduced response on the affected side.

2. Central Vertigo

Onset: Gradual, continuous, and progressive.

Symptoms: Accompanied by central nervous system signs, such as headache, papilledema, ataxia, or cranial nerve involvement.

Caloric Response: Typically symmetrical.

Causes of Peripheral Vertigo

Benign Paroxysmal Positional Vertigo (BPPV)

BPPV is a common cause of intermittent vertigo triggered by head movements. It results from displaced calcium crystals (otoliths) within the semicircular canals of the inner ear, causing inappropriate activation of the balance system. Symptoms are transient, lasting several minutes, and can recur with changes in head position. Epley's maneuver or similar repositioning exercises are effective in dislodging these crystals to less sensitive areas.

Meniere's Disease

This condition involves episodic increases in inner ear pressure, leading to damage of auditory and vestibular structures. Patients experience fluctuating hearing loss, tinnitus, and severe vertigo with nystagmus. Episodes can recur over weeks to years, with gradual residual damage. Treatment focuses on symptom management, including dietary adjustments (low-sodium diets) and medications like diuretics.

Ototoxicity

Certain medications, particularly aminoglycosides such as streptomycin and gentamicin, are toxic to the inner ear. Once vertigo, hearing loss, or tinnitus appear, the damage is often irreversible. To minimize risk, these drugs should only be used in life-threatening infections, with careful monitoring of serum levels. Discontinuation of the drug and initiation of corticosteroids (e.g., 1 mg/kg/day for 10 days) can help mitigate damage.

Vestibular Neuronitis

This condition is thought to result from inflammation of the vestibular nerve, often following a viral upper respiratory infection.

Symptoms include sudden, incapacitating vertigo that improves over weeks as the brainstem compensates. Persistent caloric deficits may occur, but recovery is typically complete with appropriate care.

Treatment and Rehabilitation

Peripheral vertigo often triggers a mismatch of sensory inputs to the brainstem, causing severe vertigo and associated symptoms like nausea and vomiting. Recovery relies on the brainstem's ability to recalibrate and compensate for the abnormal vestibular input.

1. Acute Phase Management

Medications: Labyrinthine suppressants such as dimenhydrinate or meclizine for symptom control (used sparingly for 1–2 weeks).

2. Rehabilitation

Exercises: Head movement exercises, such as nodding ("yes"), shaking ("no"), and rotation, should be performed daily. The goal is to desensitize the brainstem to triggering movements and enhance compensation.

Patients should confront, not avoid, movements that provoke symptoms to facilitate proper adaptation.

3. Compensation Process

While compensation typically occurs within weeks, it can take longer in older patients or in cases of recurrent vertigo, such as Meniere's disease. Persistent symptoms may necessitate re-evaluation to rule out central causes or other complications.

Conclusion

A systematic approach to the evaluation and management of vertigo, distinguishing between central and peripheral causes, is essential for optimizing outcomes. While peripheral vertigo often resolves with appropriate intervention, understanding the underlying mechanisms and initiating timely treatment, including rehabilitation exercises, are critical for long-term recovery.

Chapter 8
Deafness or Hearing Loss: A Comprehensive Analysis

Hearing impairment is often mistakenly perceived as a binary condition of being either fully deaf or having normal hearing. In reality, complete deafness is rare, and the term hearing loss is more appropriate, with severity measured in decibels (dB). Hearing levels range from normal (0–20 dB) to profound loss or "complete deafness" (approximately 120 dB).

Classification of Hearing Loss

1. Mild to Moderate Hearing Loss (0–60 dB):

Normal to Mild Hearing Loss (0–30 dB): This is typically within normal limits, and patients seldom report issues.

Moderate Hearing Loss (30–60 dB): Communication difficulties become noticeable, primarily for family or friends, who need to raise their voices for clarity.

2. Severe Hearing Loss (>60 dB):

Beyond 60 dB, communication challenges intensify significantly.

At levels exceeding 90–100 dB, the individual becomes functionally unable to perceive speech or sounds, making communication near-impossible without intervention.

Impact of Hearing Loss on Speech Development

Pre-Linguistic Deafness: Severe hearing loss occurring before language development (e.g., due to congenital defects or childhood meningitis) severely impairs the ability to develop normal spoken language. Rigorous training may enable partial language acquisition but is typically imperfect.

Post-Linguistic Deafness: Individuals who lose hearing after acquiring speech often experience speech deterioration due to the absence of auditory feedback.

Causes of Hearing Loss

Hearing loss may be broadly categorized into conductive and sensorineural types:

1. Conductive Hearing Loss:

This occurs when sound waves cannot reach the inner ear due to issues in the outer or middle ear, such as:

Wax buildup in the ear canal.

Middle ear fluid accumulation or infection.

Perforated eardrum.

Otosclerosis (stiffening of middle ear bones).

Conductive hearing loss generally does not exceed 50 dB because bone conduction allows sound to bypass the outer/middle ear and directly stimulate the inner ear. Although sound is reduced in intensity, its quality remains unaffected. Treatment options often include wax removal, treating infections, repairing eardrum perforations, or surgical correction of ossicle damage.

2. Sensorineural Hearing Loss:

This type results from damage to the inner ear (e.g., cochlea) or auditory pathways to the brain. It often presents with:

Tinnitus: A perceived sound, such as ringing or buzzing, caused by spontaneous inner ear impulses.

Distorted sound quality: Unlike conductive hearing loss, the clarity of sound may be impaired.

Causes include:

Aging (Presbycusis): A natural decline in auditory function.

Noise exposure: From loud music or industrial sounds.

Viral infections: Such as mumps or measles.

Drug toxicity: Aminoglycosides (e.g., gentamicin, streptomycin) and quinine compounds can induce irreversible damage.

Diagnostic Approach

Hearing loss is diagnosed using:

History and Physical Examination.

Tuning Fork Tests: Differentiate conductive from sensorineural loss:

Conductive loss is typically reversible, whereas sensorineural loss is often permanent and more severe.

Behavioral Tests: For severe hearing loss, observing patient responses to visual or auditory cues (e.g., clapping or shouting) can help gauge functional hearing levels. Note that many patients, particularly children, develop effective lip-reading skills.

Management Strategies

1. Conductive Hearing Loss:

Commonly treatable through:

Earwax removal.

Antibiotics or surgical intervention for otitis media.

Tympanoplasty for eardrum repair.

Surgical correction of ossicular chain abnormalities.

2. Sensorineural Hearing Loss:

Treatment options are limited, but early intervention may help:

Corticosteroid Therapy: A short course during the initial weeks of sudden hearing loss (e.g., 1 mg/kg/day tapered over two weeks) may partially restore hearing.

Hearing Aids: For partial loss, these devices amplify sound to improve communication.

For severe cases, particularly in children:

Early referral to specialized education programs for the deaf is critical to support language and communication skills development.

Cochlear implants may be an option for profound hearing loss in select cases.

Special Considerations

Congenital or Early-Onset Hearing Loss: May result from genetic disorders, meningitis, or ototoxic medications during childhood. Without intervention, these children face significant challenges in speech and cognitive development.

Tinnitus Management: Often associated with sensorineural loss, tinnitus can become psychologically distressing. Distraction techniques, such as listening to soothing music, may provide relief.

In conclusion, while conductive hearing loss is frequently manageable, sensorineural loss remains a more serious and often irreversible condition. Early diagnosis and tailored interventions are crucial for optimizing outcomes and preserving quality of life.

Chapter 9
Facial Paresis and Paralysis: A Detailed Analysis

Facial expression plays a crucial role in nonverbal communication. Any disruption in facial movements, such as paralysis or paresis, is not only immediately noticeable but can also cause significant social and psychological distress for the patient. Facial paralysis results from damage to the facial nerve along its extensive course through the temporal bone or its branches in the face.

Common Causes

Idiopathic Bell's Palsy: This is the most frequent cause of facial paralysis. Although its exact etiology is unclear, it is often linked to viral upper respiratory tract infections.

Iatrogenic Injury: Surgical interventions, particularly in the mastoid or middle ear, may inadvertently damage the facial nerve.

Trauma: Severe head injuries causing temporal bone fractures can lead to nerve impairment.

Infections and Inflammation: Infections in the middle ear or mastoid region, as well as viral processes, may inflame the facial nerve. In some cases, swelling within the narrow confines of the bony canal compresses the nerve's blood supply, resulting in variable nerve damage.

Herpes Zoster and Other Viral Infections

Herpes Zoster infections involving the outer ear or throat should raise suspicion of Ramsay Hunt Syndrome. This condition is associated with herpetic lesions and carries a poorer prognosis compared to Bell's palsy, with more than 50% of cases resulting in permanent damage.

Prognosis and Treatment Approaches

Bell's Palsy: This condition generally has a favorable prognosis, with over 95% of patients achieving full recovery.

Herpes Zoster-Related Paralysis: The prognosis is less favorable, and permanent deficits are more common.

Corticosteroid Therapy:
The most widely accepted treatment for idiopathic Bell's palsy is a short course of corticosteroids, which reduces inflammation and promotes recovery. A typical regimen involves administering 1 mg/kg/day in a single morning dose, gradually tapering off by 5 mg daily over two weeks. Despite the empirical nature of this treatment, it is

considered effective in many cases, with minimal adverse effects.

Surgical Intervention

Surgical decompression of the facial nerve has been suggested for traumatic or iatrogenic injuries. However, this procedure is complex and has not consistently demonstrated superior outcomes compared to conservative management.

Challenges in Management

Facial paralysis remains a challenging condition to treat, especially when neural reconstruction is required, as results are often unsatisfactory. However, spontaneous recovery is relatively common in idiopathic cases, providing hope for many patients.

Conclusion

Facial paresis and paralysis pose significant functional and social challenges. While idiopathic Bell's palsy often resolves with minimal intervention, other causes may require tailored treatment strategies. Corticosteroids remain the cornerstone of therapy for Bell's palsy, while surgical approaches are reserved for specific cases. Advances in understanding the underlying mechanisms of facial nerve damage are needed to improve treatment outcomes.

Chapter 10
Nasal Obstruction: A Detailed Overview

Nasal obstruction is among the most frequently encountered symptoms in clinical practice. Under normal conditions, airflow alternates between the nostrils due to periodic swelling of the inferior turbinates, a phenomenon known as the nasal cycle. This cycle typically occurs every 4-5 hours, where one nostril becomes partially blocked while the other facilitates breathing.

Common Causes of Nasal Obstruction

Alternating Obstruction:
Conditions such as allergic rhinitis, vasomotor rhinitis, viral rhinitis, or sinusitis often lead to increased swelling of the nasal mucosa, causing alternating nasal blockage. In children, allergic rhinitis is a common

cause, although enlarged adenoids are sometimes implicated.

Persistent Unilateral Obstruction:
Chronic blockage on one side of the nose may indicate:

Nasal Septum Deviation: A structural issue causing airflow restriction.

Foreign Body: Particularly common in pediatric cases.

Nasal Polyps or Tumors: Benign or malignant growths that obstruct the nasal passage.

Choanal Atresia: A rare congenital condition involving blockage of the nasal passage.

Symptomatology

Allergic, Vasomotor, or Viral Rhinitis:

These conditions typically present with symptoms such as watery rhinorrhea (nasal discharge) and sneezing.

Bacterial Rhinitis or Sinusitis:
Indicators include purulent nasal discharge, postnasal drip, and intermittent facial pain. These suggest infection or inflammation within the nasal and sinus passages.

Case-Based Analysis

1. Allergic Rhinitis: A patient presenting with alternating nasal obstruction, watery discharge, and sneezing likely suffers from allergic rhinitis. Management involves allergen avoidance and antihistamines.

2. Sinusitis: Complaints of unilateral obstruction with purulent discharge and facial pain point to bacterial sinusitis, warranting antibiotic therapy and nasal irrigation.

3. Nasal Polyps: Persistent unilateral blockage accompanied by anosmia (loss of smell) may suggest nasal polyps. Diagnostic confirmation via nasal endoscopy or imaging is essential.

4. Pediatric Cases: A child presenting with chronic nasal obstruction and mouth breathing may have enlarged adenoids, often coexisting with allergic rhinitis. Adenoidectomy or medical therapy may be required.

Conclusion

Nasal obstruction is a multifaceted symptom with diverse etiologies ranging from benign conditions like rhinitis to more serious causes such as tumors. Accurate diagnosis relies on a thorough history, clinical examination, and, when necessary, imaging or endoscopy. Treatment varies from conservative measures like nasal decongestants and antihistamines to surgical interventions for structural abnormalities or growths. Early identification and management are critical to alleviating symptoms and preventing complications.

Chapter 11
Sinusitis: A Comprehensive Analysis

Sinusitis refers to inflammation of the paranasal sinuses, which include the maxillary (cheek), ethmoid (between the eyes and nose), frontal (beneath the forehead), and sphenoid (beneath the hypophysis) sinuses. Any of these air-filled cavities can become involved in this condition, which often begins as a viral upper respiratory tract (URT) infection such as a cold or the flu.

Pathophysiology

The inflammatory process typically follows these stages:

1. Initiation:
Viral infections of the nasal mucosa lead to nasal obstruction and blockage of the sinus drainage pathways (ostia).

2. Formation of a Closed Cavity:
Blockage results in the isolation of the sinus cavity from external airflow. Oxygen within the cavity is absorbed by the lining tissue, causing a significant drop in pressure and creating a partial vacuum. This pressure change leads to facial and headache discomfort often associated with colds.

3. Fluid Accumulation:
Persistent low pressure induces transudate formation, while viral stimulation increases secretions. The fluid-filled cavity becomes an ideal environment for bacterial growth, leading to infection and abscess formation.

4. Clinical Symptoms:

Facial pain, particularly when bending forward.

Pain radiating to the upper molars due to proximity to the maxillary sinus.

Yellow or green nasal discharge indicating bacterial infection.

5. Chronicity:
Inflammation perpetuates the obstruction, creating a cycle that maintains the infection. Rare complications include orbital or cerebral abscess formation.

Diagnosis

Imaging:
A simple "Waters' view" X-ray, with the patient's chin against the plate, often suffices to reveal sinus fluid levels. A full sinus series is generally unnecessary unless complications arise.

Symptoms:
Sinusitis presenting with foul-smelling discharge and pus often stems from a

dental abscess involving the upper molars, commonly resulting in unilateral symptoms.

Management

1. Medical Treatment:

Antibiotics: Ampicillin or Co-Trimoxazole are commonly used but must be paired with nasal decongestants to ensure effective sinus drainage and prevent relapse.

Nasal Decongestants:

Adrenaline (1:50,000), oxymetazoline, or neosynephrine drops are recommended thrice daily for up to one month.

After one week, decongestants can be replaced with simple saline drops (boiled or distilled water).

Prolonged courses of antibiotics may be necessary for recurrent or resistant cases.

2. Surgical Intervention:

Reserved for cases where medical management fails or complications such as polyps, cysts, or inflamed mucosa obstruct the sinus permanently.

Indications include intraorbital extensions (more common in children) or intracranial complications, both of which are fortunately rare.

3. Addressing Dental Abscesses:
Sinusitis linked to a dental abscess clears after resolving the underlying dental issue.

Key Considerations

Facial swelling is not a typical symptom of sinusitis, except in rare orbital complications. If swelling occurs, it often indicates a dental abscess or tumor, necessitating further evaluation.

Most sinusitis cases respond well to conservative management, making surgery an exception rather than a routine intervention.

Conclusion

Sinusitis is a common yet multifaceted condition that requires a tailored approach based on its etiology and severity. Timely identification and treatment can prevent chronicity and rare but serious complications.

Chapter 12
Comprehensive Analysis of Headaches

Headaches are often perceived as a neurological issue; however, their causes frequently originate from otolaryngological conditions. This section provides a structured analysis of various types of headaches, focusing on their etiology, presentation, and management strategies.

Misconceptions about Headaches

Contrary to common belief, severe headaches are rarely indicative of brain tumors. Most brain tumors do not present with headaches; instead, findings like papilledema on fundoscopy are more specific. Furthermore, diagnostic imaging such as CT and MRI scans often yield negative results for primary headaches, emphasizing the importance of a thorough clinical history in diagnosis.

Common Types of Headaches

1. Idiopathic Headaches:

These are self-limiting, of unknown cause, and typically short-lived.

Symptomatic treatment is generally sufficient.

2. Migraine:

True migraines are less common and are characterized by an aura, visual disturbances (e.g., scotoma), and marked photophobia.

Management often includes identifying triggers and symptomatic relief.

3. Cluster Headaches:

Similar to migraines but lack aura or scotoma.

They occur in episodic clusters and may remain dormant for months.

Potential triggers include foods such as chocolate, coffee, or cheese.

Hormonal factors, including associations with the menstrual cycle, should be considered.

4. Sinus Headaches:

Common during the acute phase of sinusitis or initial infection.

Chronic sinusitis may cause intermittent pain.

5. Sluder Headaches:

Triggered by the nasal turbinates pressing against a deviated nasal septum or septal spur.

Diagnosed and relieved by applying a nasal anesthetic and vasoconstrictor, confirming the source of pain.

Recent studies suggest early application of nasal sprays containing lidocaine may help in migraines.

6. Cervical and Tension Headaches:

Caused by tension in cervical muscles pulling on cranial insertions or compressing occipital nerves.

Pain is localized to the occipital region and the top of the head.

Treatment includes local heat therapy or lignocaine injections, offering rapid relief.

Less Common Causes

1. Hypertension:

Rarely causes headaches but should be ruled out.

2. Neurological Conditions:

Meningitis (bacterial or viral) often presents with subtle signs of neck stiffness that must be recognized early.

Other infections, such as malaria or amoebiasis, may also manifest with headaches.

3. Structural Abnormalities:

For instance, tumors or vascular malformations, though rare, require specific diagnostic workups.

Diagnostic and Management Considerations

1. Initial Symptomatic Treatment:

Many headaches resolve with simple symptomatic care and time.

Persistent cases may require more detailed evaluation.

2. Psychological Factors:

The patient's psychological state and stress levels must be considered, as these can exacerbate symptoms or contribute to tension-type headaches.

3. Imaging and Investigations:

Imaging is reserved for cases with atypical presentations or signs of secondary headaches.

4. Parasitic Infections:

Especially in endemic areas, these should not be overlooked as potential causes.

5. Referral:

If headaches persist despite initial treatment, or if they are associated with neurological deficits or systemic symptoms, further evaluation in a specialized setting is warranted.

Conclusion

Headaches encompass a wide spectrum of causes, ranging from benign, idiopathic conditions to more serious underlying pathologies. A patient-centered approach that combines clinical history, targeted investigations, and symptomatic management is essential for effective care. The interplay of neurological, otolaryngological, and psychological factors should guide diagnosis and treatment.

Chapter 13
Hoarseness or Dysphonia: Comprehensive Analysis and Case-Based Insights

The primary function of the larynx is airway protection, with speech serving as a secondary, incidental benefit that has enabled language development and cultural evolution. Dysphonia refers broadly to any alteration in normal voice quality. This includes changes from swollen adenoids, nasal obstruction, or infections such as epiglottitis. However, clinical discussions often focus on conditions affecting the vocal cords' vibration. These causes are categorized as extralaryngeal and intralaryngeal.

Extralaryngeal Causes

Extralaryngeal factors disrupt neural control of laryngeal structures and include:

1. Psychogenic Factors
Conditions such as falsetto voice or functional aphonia fall into this category. Functional aphonia can often be differentiated by asking the patient to cough. A normal cough requires functional vocal cord closure, indicating an absence of organic disease.

2. Neurological Impairments
Neurological dysfunctions, including damage to the vagus or recurrent laryngeal nerves along their course from the brainstem to the larynx, can cause hoarseness. Coordination issues originating from the cerebellum may also contribute.

3. Neuromuscular Disorders

Diseases affecting neuromuscular transmission can impair laryngeal function and result in dysphonia.

4. Recurrent Laryngeal Nerve Damage

The recurrent laryngeal nerves are particularly vulnerable due to their long anatomical course. Damage can occur during surgeries such as thyroidectomy. The left nerve is more frequently affected because of its descent into the chest, making it susceptible to cardiovascular conditions or malignancies like bronchial carcinoma. Unilateral recurrent nerve paralysis typically results in hoarseness but does not obstruct airflow, whereas bilateral paralysis often necessitates a tracheotomy.

> Clinical Note: Any unexplained vocal cord paralysis, especially on the left, warrants a thorough investigation of the entire recurrent and vagus nerve pathway, with a particular focus on potential thoracic pathology.

Intralaryngeal Causes

Intralaryngeal causes interfere directly with the vocal cords' ability to vibrate or adduct during phonation:

1. Pubertal Voice Changes
Testosterone-induced laryngeal growth during puberty often results in temporary dysphonia ("voice breaking") in adolescent males.

2. Endocrine Disorders
Hypothyroidism affects the larynx structurally and neurologically, causing gradual voice changes. These are often first noticed by acquaintances who interact with the patient infrequently.

3. Inflammatory Conditions

Acute Causes: Conditions like acute laryngitis or upper respiratory infections.

Chronic Causes: Prolonged voice misuse, chronic infections, or smoking. Granulomatous diseases, including tuberculosis and syphilis, may also alter laryngeal structure and function.

4. Benign Lesions

Vocal Nodules: These develop due to chronic voice abuse, such as yelling or singing, and are commonly located at the junction of the anterior third and posterior two-thirds of the vocal cords. They often appear bilaterally.

Juvenile Laryngeal Papillomas: These viral lesions, linked to maternal genital condyloma at birth, manifest as progressive hoarseness and, eventually, stridor in children. Treatment involves cautious removal using electrocautery or laser while avoiding damage to laryngeal structures and preventing bleeding. Tracheotomy should be avoided due to the risk of bronchial extension.

5. Malignancies

Laryngeal Carcinoma: The most common malignant tumor of the larynx, often presenting early with hoarseness. Early diagnosis and intervention lead to favorable prognosis comparable to skin cancers. Biopsy confirmation is essential for any persistent dysphonia lasting over 6–8 weeks, especially in smokers.

Differential Diagnosis and Considerations

Dysphonia should not be confused with other speech disorders such as dysarthria (speech articulation difficulties), aphasia (language comprehension or production deficits), or apraxia (impaired motor planning of speech). Proper diagnostic differentiation is critical.

Conclusion and Clinical Recommendations

Persistent hoarseness should never be overlooked, especially in high-risk populations such as smokers or individuals with a history of thyroid surgery. Early identification of underlying conditions—whether benign or malignant—significantly improves outcomes. A systematic approach, combining clinical history, physical examination, imaging, and biopsy, ensures accurate diagnosis and effective management.

Chapter 14
Tonsillitis and Adenoids:
Comprehensive Overview

The tonsils and adenoids, along with the lingual tonsils, lymphatic follicles, and interconnecting lymphatic vessels, constitute Waldeyer's Ring. This structure forms a continuous circle of lymphoid tissue around the upper airways and food passages. Its primary function is to generate antibodies against the numerous antigens and pathogens inhaled or ingested daily, especially during early childhood. As the immune system matures and encounters fewer novel antigens, the lymphoid tissue gradually atrophies. Typically, the adenoidal tissue begins to regress after the first few years of life, followed later by the tonsils, both palatal and lingual.

Inflammation and Hypertrophy

Occasionally, this lymphoid tissue becomes inflamed or enlarged, resulting in tonsillitis or adenoiditis. The progression usually begins with a viral upper respiratory tract infection characterized by mild fever, sore throat, slight cough, and nasal discharge. Symptoms often improve after a few days, but a sudden relapse with worsening sore throat, fever, dysphagia, and general malaise may signal secondary bacterial infection. Physical examination reveals red, swollen tonsils, often with visible white exudate from the tonsillar crypts. Adenoids, although not easily observable, exhibit similar inflammatory changes.

Treatment Considerations

Tonsillitis is generally self-limiting within one to two weeks. However, severe cases can lead to fibrosis and structural changes in the tonsils, predisposing individuals to recurrent infections. Antibiotic therapy must be carefully timed and judiciously prescribed:

Initial Phase (First 3 Days): Symptomatic treatment without antibiotics is recommended during the viral stage.

Secondary Phase (After 3 Days): Antibiotics may be introduced if symptoms relapse, indicating a bacterial superinfection. A broad-spectrum antibiotic such as Co-trimoxazole, ampicillin, or a cephalosporin is typically preferred, considering the varied bacterial flora of the throat. Penicillin, although effective against β-haemolytic streptococcus, may not address other pathogens.

Antibiotics should be continued for 8-10 days, with patient reassessment after three days to determine the need for an alternative medication if no improvement is observed. Routine throat cultures are often unhelpful due to the diversity of normal bacterial flora.

Surgical Indications

Surgery is reserved for cases of recurrent or severe tonsillitis. Criteria for tonsillectomy typically include more than five severe episodes per year. Tonsillar size alone is not a reliable indicator; instead, the degree of hyperemia in the anterior tonsillar pillars is more informative. Adenoidectomy is warranted when hypertrophic adenoids cause significant obstruction of nasal respiration, although nasal turbinate issues are often a more common cause of nasal obstruction.

Clinical Assessment of Adenoidal Obstruction

Adenoidal size can be evaluated using lateral neck X-rays or laryngeal mirrors. A simple clinical method involves assessing soft palate mobility with tongue depressors. If the difference in mobility is less than 5 mm (normal range: 8–10 mm), it suggests significant obstruction.

Surgical Procedure

Tonsillectomy and adenoidectomy are typically performed under general anesthesia. The tonsils are carefully dissected from the surrounding mucosa, with bleeding vessels ligated or cauterized. Enlarged adenoids, if present, are removed simultaneously using an adenoid curette. While tonsillitis itself is not life-threatening, the surgical procedure poses risks, including severe hemorrhage or airway compromise. Consequently, it should be conducted by a specialist or under close supervision.

In conclusion, while tonsillitis and adenoiditis are common conditions, their management requires a balance between conservative and surgical approaches, guided by the severity and frequency of infections. Judicious use of antibiotics and careful consideration of surgical indications ensure optimal outcomes while minimizing risks.

Chapter 15
Tumors in the Neck and Thyroid Nodules: Clinical Approach and Management

Neck Tumors

A persistent neck mass should be regarded as potentially malignant until proven otherwise. Initial management involves ruling out infectious causes by prescribing a short course of broad-spectrum antibiotics and performing a Mantoux test. If these yield negative results, fine-needle aspiration biopsy (FNAB) is recommended over excisional biopsy to avoid compromising subsequent treatment protocols.

FNAB represents a significant advancement in managing neck tumors. It is minimally invasive, requires no anesthesia, and is cost-effective. Additionally, the risk of needle-tract metastasis is exceedingly low.

A proficient cytologist or pathologist is essential for interpreting the biopsy results, which can be easily sent for remote analysis. This procedure is straightforward and highly effective when performed correctly, contributing to accurate diagnoses without unnecessary surgical risks.

Thyroid Nodules

Thyroid nodules are unique among neck tumors due to their prevalence and relatively low malignancy rates—less than 20% in solitary nodules and under 10% in multinodular goiters. Conducting unnecessary thyroidectomies on all nodules is not justified. However, distinguishing between benign and malignant nodules often relies on clinical expertise, as no single diagnostic tool guarantees accuracy.

Clinical Features Suggestive of Malignancy:

1. Recent changes in the nodule's size, shape, or texture, particularly increased hardness or fixation.

2. Presence of lymphadenopathy, especially involving jugulo-omohyoid nodes.

3. Symptoms such as hoarseness, difficulty swallowing, or breathing (dysphonia, dysphagia, stridor).

4. Family history of thyroid disorders or malignancy.

5. Patient demographics:

Age <20 years (50% of thyroid nodules in children are malignant).

Age >65 years, particularly in males.

Diagnostic Investigations

Thyroid function tests typically remain normal in cases of thyroid nodules, limiting their diagnostic utility. Thyroid scintigraphy can help differentiate "hot" (functioning) nodules from "cold" (non-functioning) ones, but it may not provide conclusive evidence of malignancy. Cold nodules, including cystic ones, require further evaluation with FNAB to confirm their nature.

Fine-Needle Aspiration Biopsy (FNAB):
FNAB serves as both a diagnostic and therapeutic tool, especially for cystic lesions. Small cysts are infrequently malignant and can often be managed with repeated aspiration and observation. In contrast, large cystic nodules typically warrant surgical excision.

Management Strategies

Observation and Medical Management:

Small nodules and cysts may be treated with thyroid suppression therapy using thyroxine and closely monitored for changes.

Surgical Intervention:
Surgery is indicated for nodules exhibiting suspicious characteristics or those falling within high-risk categories. In such cases, a thyroid lobectomy is performed, and the excised tissue is sent for pathological analysis.

Surgical Considerations:
When deciding between partial, subtotal, or total thyroidectomy, it is crucial to minimize risks to vital structures:

Protect the recurrent laryngeal nerves to avoid vocal cord paralysis.

Preserve at least one functioning parathyroid gland to prevent hypoparathyroidism, which is more challenging to manage than thyroid hormone deficiency.

Post-thyroidectomy, hormone replacement with levothyroxine effectively manages hypothyroidism, ensuring a good quality of life for the patient.

Key Takeaways

The management of neck tumors and thyroid nodules requires a judicious blend of clinical acumen, minimally invasive diagnostic tools, and thoughtful surgical intervention. FNAB remains a cornerstone of diagnosis, while surgical decisions should prioritize preserving function and minimizing complications.

Chapter 16
Nasal Fractures: Diagnosis and Management

Diagnosis

The diagnosis of a nasal fracture is primarily clinical and does not require imaging such as X-rays. fractures typically do not necessitate surgical intervention. Due to the thin skin and mucosal layers covering the nasal bones, clinical examination is usually sufficient to identify fractures. Particular attention should be given to the nasal septum, as displacement is common following trauma.

Timing of Intervention

Reduction or realignment of nasal fractures should ideally occur within a week of the injury, though earlier intervention often yields better outcomes.

Septal Hematoma and Its Risks

A critical complication of nasal trauma is a septal hematoma, which presents as a rounded swelling within the nasal cavity, often causing complete nasal obstruction. Left untreated, the hematoma can become infected, leading to the formation of an abscess. This can destroy the septal cartilage, causing nasal deformities such as saddle nose. Additionally, due to shared venous drainage, there is a risk of intracranial complications.

Treatment for Septal Hematoma:

Aspiration or Incision: A large needle or a 1 cm mucosal incision can drain the hematoma or abscess.

Nasal Packing: Packing the nose prevents reaccumulation of blood.

Evaluation of Severe Facial Trauma

In cases of significant facial trauma, carefully palpate the orbital rims and check for movement of the upper teeth and palate to identify potential facial fractures. These fractures often align with the Le Fort classification (I, II, or III), based on predictable fracture patterns.

Management of Nasal Fractures

1. Preparation:

Place the patient in a supine position.

Pack the nasal cavity with cotton wool soaked in 10% xylocaine spray and oxymetazoline drops. Ensure the packing reaches under the nasal bones and into the nasal vault.

Administer 2% xylocaine with epinephrine (1:200,000) via an insulin syringe to anesthetize the infraorbital, supratrochlear, infratrochlear nerves, and external nasal branches.

2. Anesthesia Application:

Wait approximately 15 minutes for the anesthesia to take effect.

Test the area with a needle and apply additional anesthetic if necessary.

3. Fracture Reduction:

Remove the nasal pack and replace it with gauze between the septum and inferior turbinate to prevent blood drainage into the throat.

Gently massage the nasal dorsum to reduce swelling and locate the fracture line.

Reduce the fracture using simple manual pressure; specialized instruments are not usually required. Avoid using forceps like Welsham's or Asche's, which can exacerbate bruising and bleeding.

For depressed nasal bones, elevate them using straight Mayo scissors inserted under the nasal vault.

4. Septal Realignment:

Assess and correct the septal position as needed using Mayo scissors.

5. Stabilization:

If the fracture is unstable, pack the nasal cavity with gauze strips to stabilize both the nasal dorsum and septum internally.

Externally tape the nose to minimize edema and apply a plaster of Paris splint for additional stabilization.

6. Post-Procedure Care:

Remove internal packing after 2-3 days, depending on the stability of the fracture.

Retain the splint for 5 days and use micropore tape for up to 2 weeks to maintain alignment and support.

Key Considerations

Proper handling of nasal fractures ensures optimal outcomes and minimizes complications. Early intervention, careful reduction techniques, and vigilant monitoring for septal hematomas are essential components of effective management.

Chapter 17
Dysphagia: Assessment and Management

Definition and Significance

Dysphagia, the difficulty or inability to swallow effectively, is a significant clinical symptom that requires thorough evaluation. It can indicate various underlying conditions ranging from structural abnormalities to neurological disorders.

Key Diagnostic Considerations

1. Differentiating Solids vs. Liquids:

Easier swallowing of liquids than solids:
This pattern suggests structural issues such as:

Carcinoma or strictures: Evaluate for associated symptoms like a history of gastric reflux, achalasia, or prior ingestion of foreign objects, caustic substances, or acids (whether accidental or intentional).

More difficulty swallowing liquids than solids:
This indicates a swallowing coordination issue, typically linked to neurological conditions.

2. Sensation of a Lump in the Throat:

A painless "lump" felt during swallowing without obstruction may result from a cricopharyngeal muscle spasm at the esophageal entrance, often due to anxiety or neurosis.

3. Painful Swallowing (Odynophagia):

Conditions causing severe pain during swallowing include:

Severe tonsillitis

Peritonsillar abscess

Pharyngitis

Retropharyngeal abscess

Epiglottitis

In these cases, the swallowing difficulty arises from pain rather than a physical or functional blockage.

Diagnostic Approach for Persistent Dysphagia

Duration: Persistent symptoms lasting several weeks necessitate advanced investigation.

Diagnostic Tools:

Barium Swallow: Provides imaging to assess structural abnormalities.

Endoscopy: Direct visualization of the esophagus, including biopsies of any suspicious areas, is essential for identifying malignancies or other pathological changes.

Summary

A systematic approach to dysphagia involves differentiating between structural and functional causes, recognizing associated symptoms, and conducting appropriate imaging and endoscopic evaluations. Early and accurate diagnosis is vital to managing the underlying condition effectively.

Chapter 18
Language and Speech Challenges in Children: A Clinical Overview

Significance of Language in Development

Language is fundamental to human cognition and social interaction. It enables rational thinking, planning, and contemplation of past and future events, distinguishing humans from other species.

Speech Development in Children

1. Typical Milestones:

Most children begin developing speech around their first birthday, with girls often starting earlier than boys.

Research indicates that children with an IQ above 60 generally acquire speech.

2. Innate Language Acquisition:

Humans possess an inherent drive to communicate, and even isolated groups can create and use a language.

Before the age of 10–12, children can learn any language fluently and without an accent. This period is crucial for auditory and linguistic development.

3. Impact of Secretory Otitis Media:

Many children experience secretory otitis media during critical developmental years. This condition, which impairs auditory input, can significantly hinder language acquisition.

Delayed Language Development

If a child has not started developing language by age two, a comprehensive evaluation is necessary to identify underlying causes.

Components of Verbal Communication

Language development involves a complex integration of several processes:

1. Reception (Hearing): Functioning of the ears and auditory system.

2. Perception (Auditory Processing): Understanding and interpreting sounds.

3. Integration (Cognition): Higher cerebral functions that synthesize auditory and conceptual inputs.

4. Expression (Speech Production): Mechanisms for producing spoken language.

5. Voice (Laryngeal Function): Functionality of the larynx for vocalization.

Each step must be systematically assessed when speech delays are observed.

Diagnostic Approach

1. Hearing Assessment:

Conditions like secretory otitis media can cause hearing loss severe enough to delay speech development.

2. Tongue Tie Misconceptions:

Contrary to popular belief, tongue tie (short frenulum) rarely contributes to speech issues.

Conclusion

Early identification and intervention are essential for addressing language and speech delays in children. A methodical approach to assessing auditory, cognitive, and speech production processes can help ensure timely support and optimal development.

References

1. Adams, R. D., & Victor, M. (Eds.). (2009). Principles of Neurology (9th ed.). McGraw-Hill Education.

2. Bailey, B. J., & Johnson, J. T. (Eds.). (2014). Head and Neck Surgery – Otolaryngology (5th ed.). Lippincott Williams & Wilkins.

3. Berkowitz, R. G., & Hannington, H. (2016). Essential Otolaryngology: Head and Neck Surgery (12th ed.). McGraw-Hill Education.

4. Bhattacharyya, N. (2016). The role of nasal and sinus disease in chronic respiratory disease. Otolaryngology–Head and Neck Surgery, 154(3), 481-486.

5. Bluestone, C. D., & Gates, G. A. (Eds.). (2019). Pediatric Otolaryngology (5th ed.). Elsevier.

6. Brook, I. (2014). Chronic Sinusitis: A Practical Guide. Springer.

7. Chandler, J. R., & Karmody, C. S. (2017). Otolaryngology: A Short Course. Wiley-Blackwell.

8. Cummings, C. W., Flint, P. W., Haughey, B. H., & Thomas, J. R. (Eds.). (2015). Cummings Otolaryngology: Head and Neck Surgery (6th ed.). Elsevier.

9. Dagan, R. (2017). Infections of the Upper Respiratory Tract and Otolaryngology. Elsevier.

10. Dykeman, K., & Dufresne, D. (2016). Practical Guide to Ear, Nose, and Throat Disorders. Springer.

11. Harrison, T. R., & Kasper, D. L. (Eds.). (2018). Harrison's Principles of Internal Medicine (20th ed.). McGraw-Hill Education.

12. Harter, P., & McCaffrey, T. V. (2017). Caring for the Patient with Throat Disorders. Elsevier.

13. Kacprzak, M. (2014). Surgical Techniques in Otolaryngology: Head and Neck Surgery. Springer.

14. Lanza, D. C., & Kennedy, D. W. (2014). Adult and Pediatric Otolaryngology: Head and Neck Surgery. Elsevier.

15. Lanza, D. C., & Kennedy, D. W. (2016). Endoscopic Sinus Surgery: Anatomy, Technique, and Complications. Elsevier.

16. Laryngology and Otology Section, American Academy of Otolaryngology–Head and Neck Surgery.

(2018). Principles of Otolaryngology: A Guide for Clinicians. Elsevier.

17. Marchese, R. R., & Rivas, M. J. (2017). Ear, Nose, and Throat Emergencies: A Practical Approach. Springer.

18. Miller, R. D., & Pardo, M. C. (Eds.). (2019). Anesthesia for Otolaryngologic Surgery. Elsevier.

19. Nardone, R. (2016). Otolaryngology and Its Disorders. McGraw-Hill Education.

20. Pracy, P., & Powell, S. (2012). Surgical Techniques in Head and Neck Surgery and Oncology. Wiley-Blackwell.

21. Proctor, T. (2013). The Complete ENT Examination and Diagnosis: A Practical Guide. Springer.

22. Sataloff, R. T. (Ed.). (2017). Professional Voice: The Science and Art of Clinical Care (4th ed.). Plural Publishing.

23. Shields, T. W. (2006). General Thoracic Surgery (7th ed.). Lippincott Williams & Wilkins.

24. Young, M., & Robinson, M. (2015). Otolaryngology: A Clinical Handbook. Springer.

www.ingramcontent.com/pod-product-compliance
Lightning Source LLC
Chambersburg PA
CBHW071025240526
45469CB00006BD/2101